# The Essential Keto Diet Cookbook

Easy and Delicious Ketogenic Recipes to Boost Your Metabolism and Lose Weight Fast

## Allison Rivera

# Table Of Content

# SMOOTHIES & BREAKFAST

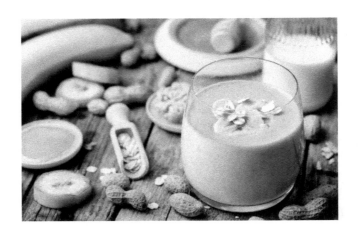

# Cinnamon Coconut

# Smoothie

Preparation Time: 5 minutes Cooking Time: 5

minutes Serve: 1

## Ingredients:

- 1/2 tsp cinnamon
- 1 scoop vanilla protein powder
- 1 tbsp shredded coconut
- 3/4 cup unsweetened almond milk
- 1/4 cup unsweetened coconut milk

## Directions:

1. Add all ingredients into the blender and blend until smooth.
2. Serve and enjoy.

## Nutritional Value (Amount per Serving):

Calories 300

Fat 18.7 g

Carbohydrates 5 g

Sugar 2.6 g

Protein 29.3 g

Cholesterol 2 mg

# Lemon Chaffle

Preparation Time: 10 minutes

Cooking Time: 12 minutes

Servings: 3-4

## Ingredients:

- 1 egg
- ¼ cup mozzarella cheese, shredded
- 1 oz. cream cheese
- 2 teaspoons lemon juice
- 2 tablespoons sweetener
- 1 teaspoon baking powder
- 4 tablespoons almond flour

## Method:

1. Preheat your waffle maker.
2. Beat the egg in a bowl.
3. Stir in the two cheeses.
4. Add the remaining ingredients.
5. Mix well.
6. Pour batter into the waffle maker.
7. Cook for 4 minutes.
8. Open and let waffle cook for 2 minutes.
9. Add the remaining batter to the device and repeat the steps.

## Nutritional Value:

- Calories 166
- Total Fat 9.5g
- Saturated Fat 4.3g
- Cholesterol 99mg
- Sodium 99mg
- Potassium 305mg
- Total Carbohydrate 3.7g
- Dietary Fiber 1g
- Protein 5.6g

# Nut Butter Chaffle

Preparation Time: 10 minutes

Cooking Time: 8 minutes

Servings: 2

## Ingredients:

- 1 egg
- ½ cup mozzarella cheese, shredded
- 2 tablespoons almond flour
- ½ teaspoon baking powder
- 1 tablespoon sweetener
- 1 teaspoon vanilla
- 2 tablespoons nut butter

## Method:

1. Turn on the waffle maker.
2. Beat the egg in a bowl and combine with the cheese.
3. In another bowl, mix the almond flour, baking powder and sweetener.
4. In the third bowl, blend the vanilla extract and nut butter.
5. Gradually add the almond flour mixture into the egg mixture.
6. Then, stir in the vanilla extract.
7. Pour the batter into the waffle maker.
8. Cook for 4 minutes.
9. Transfer to a plate and let cool for 2 minutes.
10. Repeat the steps with the remaining batter.

## Nutritional Value:

- Calories 168
- Total Fat 15.5g
- Saturated Fat 3.9g
- Cholesterol 34mg
- Sodium 31mg
- Potassium 64mg
- Total Carbohydrate 1.6g
- Dietary Fiber 1.4g
- Protein 5.4g
- Total Sugars 0.6g

# Pizza Flavored

# Chaffle

Preparation Time: 10 minutes

Cooking Time: 12 minutes

Servings: 3

## Ingredients:

- 1 egg, beaten
- ½ cup cheddar cheese, shredded
- 2 tablespoons pepperoni, chopped
- 1 tablespoon keto marinara sauce
- 4 tablespoons almond flour
- 1 teaspoon baking powder
- ½ teaspoon dried Italian seasoning
- Parmesan cheese, grated

## Method:

1. Preheat your waffle maker.
2. In a bowl, mix the egg, cheddar cheese, pepperoni, marinara sauce, almond flour, baking powder and Italian seasoning.
3. Add the mixture to the waffle maker.
4. Close the device and cook for 4 minutes.
5. Open it and transfer chaffle to a plate.
6. Let cool for 2 minutes.
7. Repeat the steps with the remaining batter.
8. Top with the grated Parmesan and serve.

## Nutritional Value:

- Calories 179
- Total Fat 14.3g
- Saturated Fat 7.5g
- Cholesterol 118mg
- Sodium 300mg
- Potassium 326mg
- Total Carbohydrate 1.8g
- Dietary Fiber 0.1g
- Protein 11.1g
- Total Sugars 0.4g

# Banana Nut Muffin

Preparation Time: 10 minutes

Cooking Time: 12 minutes

Servings: 3-4

## Ingredients:

- 1 egg
- 1 oz. cream cheese
- ¼ cup mozzarella cheese, shredded
- 1 teaspoon banana extract
- 2 tablespoons sweetener
- 1 teaspoon baking powder
- 4 tablespoons almond flour
- 2 tablespoons walnuts, chopped

## Method:

1. Combine all the ingredients in a bowl.
2. Turn on the waffle maker.
3. Add the batter to the waffle maker.
4. Seal and cook for 4 minutes.
5. Open and transfer the waffle to a plate. Let cool for 2 minutes.
6. Do the same steps with the remaining mixture.

## Nutritional Value:

- Calories 169
- Total Fat 14g
- Saturated Fat 4.6g

- Cholesterol 99mg

- Sodium 98mg

- Potassium 343mg

- Total Carbohydrate 5.6g

- Dietary Fiber 2g

- Protein 7.5g

Total Sugars 0.6g

# Chocolate Chaffle

Preparation Time: 5 minutes

Cooking Time: 8 minutes

Servings: 2

**Ingredients:**

- 1 egg
- ½ cup mozzarella cheese, shredded
- ½ teaspoon baking powder
- 2 tablespoons cocoa powder
- 2 tablespoons sweetener
- 2 tablespoons almond flour

**Method:**

1. Turn your waffle maker on.
2. Beat the egg in a bowl.
3. Stir in the rest of the ingredients.
4. Put the mixture into the waffle maker.
5. Seal the device and cook for 4 minutes.
6. Open and transfer the chaffle to a plate to cool for 2 minutes.
7. Do the same steps using the remaining mixture.

**Nutritional Value:**

- Calories 149
- Total Fat 10.8g
- Saturated Fat 2.4g
- Cholesterol 86mg

- Sodium 80mg
- Potassium 291mg
- Total Carbohydrate 9g
- Dietary Fiber 4.1g
- Protein 8.8g
- Total Sugars 0.3g

# Maple Syrup & Vanilla Chaffle

Preparation Time: 10 minutes

Cooking Time: 12 minutes

Servings: 3

## Ingredients:

- 1 egg, beaten
- ¼ cup mozzarella cheese, shredded
- 1 oz. cream cheese
- 1 teaspoon vanilla
- 1 tablespoon keto maple syrup
- 1 teaspoon sweetener
- 1 teaspoon baking powder
- 4 tablespoons almond flour

## Method:

1. Preheat your waffle maker.
2. Add all the ingredients to a bowl.
3. Mix well.
4. Pour some of the batter into the waffle maker.
5. Cover and cook for 4 minutes.
6. Transfer chaffle to a plate and let cool for 2 minutes.
7. Repeat the same process with the remaining mixture.

## Nutritional Value:

- Calories 146
- Total Fat 9.5g
- Saturated Fat 4.3g
- Cholesterol 99mg
- Potassium 322mg
- Sodium 99mg
- Total Carbohydrate 10.6g
- Dietary Fiber 0.9g
- Protein 5.6g
- Total Sugars 6.4g

# Chaffle Tortilla

Preparation Time: 5 minutes

Cooking Time: 8 minutes

Servings: 2

## Ingredients:

- 1 egg
- ½ cup cheddar cheese, shredded
- 1 teaspoon baking powder
- 4 tablespoons almond flour
- ¼ teaspoon garlic powder
- 1 tablespoon almond milk
- Homemade salsa
- Sour cream
- Jalapeno pepper, chopped

**Method:**

1. Preheat your waffle maker.

2. Beat the egg in a bowl.

3. Stir in the cheese, baking powder, flour, garlic powder and almond milk.

4. Pour half of the batter into the waffle maker.

5. Cover and cook for 4 minutes.

6. Open and transfer to a plate. Let cool for 2 minutes.

7. Do the same for the remaining batter.

8. Top the waffle with salsa, sour cream and jalapeno pepper.

9. Roll the waffle.

**Nutritional Value:**

- Calories 225
- Total Fat 17.6g
- Saturated Fat 9.9g
- Cholesterol 117mg
- Sodium 367mg
- Potassium 366mg
- Total Carbohydrate 6g
- Dietary Fiber 0.8g
- Protein 11.3g
- Total Sugars 1.9g

# Churro Chaffle

Preparation Time: 5 minutes

Cooking Time: 8 minutes

Servings: 2

## Ingredients:

- 1 egg
- ½ cup mozzarella cheese, shredded
- ½ teaspoon cinnamon
- 2 tablespoons sweetener

## Method:

1. Turn on your waffle iron.
2. Beat the egg in a bowl.
3. Stir in the cheese.
4. Pour half of the mixture into the waffle maker.
5. Cover the waffle iron.
6. Cook for 4 minutes.
7. While waiting, mix the cinnamon and sweetener in a bowl.
8. Open the device and soak the waffle in the cinnamon mixture.
9. Repeat the steps with the remaining batter.

## Nutritional Value:

- Calories 106
- Total Fat 6.9g
- Saturated Fat 2.9g
- Cholesterol 171mg
- Sodium 147mg
- Potassium 64mg
- Total Carbohydrate 5.8g
- Dietary Fiber 2.6g
- Protein 9.6g
- Total Sugars 0.4g

# Chocolate Chip

# Chaffle

Preparation Time: 5 minutes

Cooking Time: 8 minutes

Servings: 2

**Ingredients:**

- 1 egg
- ½ teaspoon coconut flour
- ¼ teaspoon baking powder
- 1 teaspoon sweetener
- 1 tablespoon heavy whipping cream
- 1 tablespoon chocolate chips

**Method:**

1. Preheat your waffle maker.
2. Beat the egg in a bowl.
3. Stir in the flour, baking powder, sweetener and cream.
4. Pour half of the mixture into the waffle maker.
5. Sprinkle the chocolate chips on top and close.
6. Cook for 4 minutes.
7. Remove the chaffle and put on a plate.
8. Do the same procedure with the remaining batter.

## Nutritional Value:

- Calories 146
- Total Fat 10 g
- Saturated Fat 7 g
- Cholesterol 88 mg
- Sodium 140 mg
- Potassium 50 mg
- Total Carbohydrate 5 g
- Dietary Fiber 3 g
- Protein 6 g
- Total Sugars 1 g

# Red Velvet Chaffle

Preparation Time: 5 minutes

Cooking Time: 12 minutes

Servings: 3

**Ingredients:**

- 1 egg
- ¼ cup mozzarella cheese, shredded
- 1 oz. cream cheese
- 4 tablespoons almond flour
- 1 teaspoon baking powder
- 2 teaspoons sweetener
- 1 teaspoon red velvet extract
- 2 tablespoons cocoa powder

**Method:**

1. Combine all the ingredients in a bowl.
2. Plug in your waffle maker.
3. Pour some of the batter into the waffle maker.
4. Seal and cook for 4 minutes.
5. Open and transfer to a plate.
6. Repeat the steps with the remaining batter.

## Nutritional Value:

- Calories 126
- Total Fat 10.1g
- Saturated Fat 3.4g
- Cholesterol 66mg
- Sodium 68mg
- Potassium 290mg
- Total Carbohydrate 6.5g
- Dietary Fiber 2.8g
- Protein 5.9g
- Total Sugars 0.2g

# Asparagus Pesto Chicken

Preparation Time: 10 minutes Cooking Time: 15 minutes Serve: 3

## Ingredients:

- 1 lb chicken thighs, skinless, boneless, and cut into pieces
- 3/4 lb asparagus, trimmed and cut in half
- 2 tbsp olive oil
- 1 3/4 cups grape tomatoes, halved
- 1/4 cup basil pesto
- Pepper
- Salt

## Directions:

1. Heat oil in a pan over medium heat.
2. Add chicken to the pan and season
3. with pepper and salt and cook for 5-8 minutes.
4. Add pesto and asparagus and cook for 2-3 minutes.
5. Remove pan from heat and add tomatoes and stir well.
6. Serve and enjoy.

## Nutritional Value (Amount per Serving):

Calories 415

Fat 21 g

Carbohydrates 10 g

Sugar 5 g

Protein 48 g

Cholesterol 136 mg

# PORK, BEEF & LAMB RECIPES

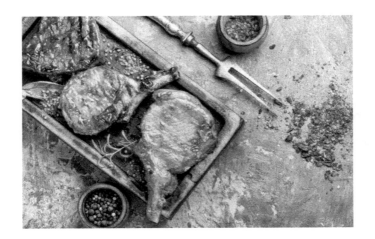

# Stuff Cheese Pork Chops

Preparation Time: 10 minutes Cooking Time: 25 minutes

Serve: 4

## Ingredients:

- 4 pork chops, boneless and thick cut
- 2 tbsp olives, chopped
- 2 tbsp sun-dried tomatoes, chopped
- ½ cup feta cheese, crumbled
- 2 garlic cloves, minced
- 2 tbsp fresh parsley, chopped

## Directions:

1. Preheat the oven to 375 F.
2. In a bowl, mix together feta cheese, garlic, parsley, olives, and sun-dried tomatoes.
3. Stuff feta cheese mixture in the pork chops. Season with pepper and salt.
4. Bake for 35 minutes.
5. Serve and enjoy.

## Nutritional Value (Amount per Serving):

Calories 316

Fat 25 g

Carbohydrates 2 g

Sugar 1 g

Protein 21 g

Cholesterol 75 mg

# Onion Paprika Pork Tenderloin

Preparation Time: 10 minutes Cooking Time: 30 minutes Serve: 6

**Ingredients:**

- 2 lbs pork tenderloin
- For rub:
- 1 1/2 tbsp smoked paprika
- 1 tbsp garlic powder
- 1 1/2 tbsp onion powder
- ½ tbsp salt

**Directions:**

1. Preheat the oven to 425 F.
2. In a small bowl, mix together all rub ingredients and rub over pork tenderloin.
3. Spray pan with cooking spray and heat over medium-high heat.
4. Sear pork on all sides until lightly golden brown.
5. Place pan into the oven and roast for about 25-30 minutes.
6. Sliced and serve.

**Nutritional Value (Amount per Serving):**

Calories 225

Fat 5 g

Carbohydrates 2 g

Sugar 1 g

Protein 41 g

Cholesterol 45 mg

# SEAFOOD & FISH RECIPES

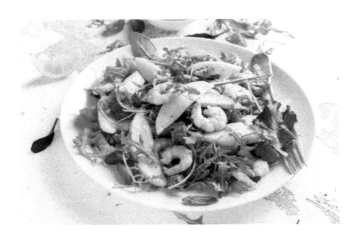

# Smooth Broccoli Cauliflower Mashed

Preparation Time: 10 minutes Cooking Time: 10 minutes Serve: 4

## Ingredients:

- 2 cups cauliflower florets
- 2 cups broccoli florets
- 2 garlic cloves, peeled
- ¼ tsp onion powder
- 1 tbsp olive oil
- 1/2 tsp pepper
- 1/2 tsp salt

## Directions:

1. Heat olive oil in a pan over medium heat.
2. Add cauliflower, broccoli, and salt in a pan and sauté until softened.
3. Transfer vegetables and garlic to the food processor and process until smooth.
4. Season with onion powder, pepper and salt.
5. Serve and enjoy.

## Nutritional Value (Amount per Serving):

Calories 60

Fat 3 g

Carbohydrates 6 g

Sugar 2 g

Protein 2 g

Cholesterol 0 mg

# Tilapia with Herbed Butter

Serves: 6

Prep Time: 35 mins

Ingredients

- 2 pounds tilapia fillets
- 12 garlic cloves, chopped finely
- 6 green broccoli, chopped
- 2 cups herbed butter
- Salt and black pepper, to taste

Directions

1. Season the tilapia fillets with salt and black pepper.
2. Put the seasoned tilapia along with all other ingredients in an Instant Pot and mix well.
3. Cover the lid and cook on High Pressure for about 25 minutes.
4. Dish out in a platter and serve hot.

Nutrition Amount per serving

Calories 281

Total Fat 10.4g 13% Saturated Fat 4.3g 21% Cholesterol 109mg 36%

Sodium 178mg 8%

Total Carbohydrate 9g 3%

Dietary Fiber 2.5g 9% Total Sugars 1.9g

Protein 38.7g

# Roasted Trout

Serves: 4

- ½ cup fresh lemon juice

- 1 pound trout fish fillets

- 4 tablespoons butter

- Salt and black pepper, to taste

- 1 teaspoon dried rosemary, crushed

Directions

1. Put ½ pound trout fillets in a dish and sprinkle with lemon juice and dried rosemary.
2. Season with salt and black pepper and transfer into a skillet.
3. Add butter and cook, covered on medium low heat for about 35 minutes.
4. Dish out the fillets in a platter and serve with a sauce.

Nutrition Amount per serving

Calories 349

Total Fat 28.2g 36% Saturated Fat 11.7g 58%

Cholesterol 31mg  10%

Sodium 88mg 4%

Total Carbohydrate 1.1g 0%

Dietary Fiber 0.3g  1%

Total Sugars 0.9g

Protein 23.3g

# Sour Fish with Herbed Butter

Serves: 3

- 2 tablespoons herbed butter

- 3 cod fillets

- 1 tablespoon vinegar

- Salt and black pepper, to taste

- ½ tablespoon lemon pepper seasoning

Directions

1. Preheat the oven to 3750F and grease a baking tray.
2. Mix together cod fillets, vinegar, lemon pepper seasoning, salt and black pepper in a bowl.
3. Marinate for about 3 hours and then arrange on the baking tray.
4. Transfer into the oven and bake for about 30 minutes.
5. Remove from the oven and serve with herbed butter.

Nutrition Amount per serving

Calories 234

Total Fat 11.8g 15%

Saturated Fat 2.4g 12%

Cholesterol 77mg 26%

Sodium 119mg 5%

Total Carbohydrate 0.4g 0%

Dietary Fiber 0g 0%

Total Sugars 0.1g

Protein 31.5g

# Cod Coconut Curry

Serves: 6

Prep Time: 35 mins

Ingredients

- 1 onion, chopped

- 2 pounds cod

- 1 cup dry coconut, chopped

- Salt and black pepper, to taste

- 1 cup fresh lemon juice

Directions

1. Put the cod along with all other ingredients in a pressure cooker.
2. Add 2 cups of water and cover the lid.
3. Cook on High Pressure for about 25 minutes and naturally release the pressure.
4. Open the lid and dish out the curry to serve hot.

Nutrition Amount per serving

Calories 223 To-

tal Fat 6.1g 8%

Saturated Fat 4.5g 23%

Cholesterol 83mg 28%

Sodium 129mg 6%

Total Carbohydrate 4.6g 2%

Dietary Fiber 1.8g 6%

Total Sugars 2.5g

Protein 35.5g

# Baked Salmon

Preparation Time: 10 minutes Cooking Time: 35 minutes

Serve: 4

## Ingredients:

- 1 lb salmon fillet
- 4 tbsp parsley, chopped
- 1/4 cup mayonnaise
- 1/4 cup parmesan cheese, grated
- 2 garlic cloves, minced
- 2 tbsp butter

## Directions:

1. Preheat the oven to 350 F.
2. Place salmon on greased baking tray.
3. Melt butter in a pan over medium heat.
4. Add garlic and sauté for minute.
5. Add remaining ingredient and stir to combined.
6. Spread pan mixture over salmon fillet.
7. Bake for 20-25 minutes.
8. Serve and enjoy.

## Nutritional Value (Amount per Serving):

Calories 412

Protein 34 g

Fat 26 g

Cholesterol 99 mg

Carbohydrates 4.3 g

Sugar 1 g

# MEATLESS MEALS

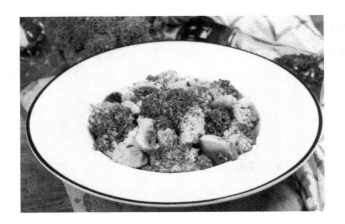

# Cauliflower Mash

Preparation Time: 10 minutes  Cooking Time: 10 minutes

Serve: 4

**Ingredients:**

- 1 lb cauliflower, cut into florets
- 1 tbsp lemon juice
- ¼ tsp onion powder
- 3 oz parmesan cheese, grated
- 4 oz butter
- ½ tsp garlic powder
- Pepper
- Salt

**Directions:**

1. Boil cauliflower florets until tender. Drain well.
2. Add cooked cauliflower into the blender with remaining ingredients and blend until smooth.
3. Serve and enjoy.

**Nutritional Value (Amount per Serving):**

Calories 300

Fat 28 g

Carbohydrates 7 g

Sugar 3 g

Protein 10 g

Cholesterol 75 mg

# SOUPS, STEWS
# & SALADS

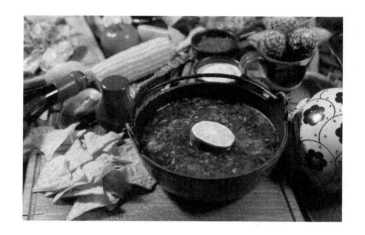

# Easy Mexican

# Chicken Soup

Preparation Time: 10 minutes Cooking Time: 4 hours

Serve: 6

## Ingredients:

- 8 oz pepper jack cheese, shredded
- 14.5 oz chicken stock
- 14 oz salsa
- 2 lbs chicken, boneless and skinless
- Pepper
- Salt

## Directions:

1. Add all ingredients into the slow cooker and stir well.
2. Cover and cook on high for 4 hours.
3. Remove chicken from slow cooker and shred using fork.
4. Return shredded chicken to the slow cooker and stir well.
5. Serve and enjoy.

**Nutritional Value (Amount per Serving):**

Calories 330

Fat 23 g

Carbohydrates 4 g

Sugar 3 g

Protein 24 g

Cholesterol 90 mg

# APPETIZERS & DESSERTS

## Pepper Jack

## Brussels Sprouts

Serves: 9

Prep Time: 20 mins

### Ingredients

- 2 pounds Brussels sprouts, halved and boiled
- 2 tablespoons garlic, minced
- 3 cups pepper jack cheese, shredded
- 2 tablespoons coconut oil
- 1 cup sour cream

### Directions

1. Heat oil in a skillet on medium heat and add garlic.
2. Sauté for about 1 minute and stir in the sour cream and pepper jack cheese.
3. Cook for about 5 minutes on medium low heat and add Brussels sprouts.
4. Stir to coat well and cover with the lid.
5. Cook for about 5 minutes and dish out into a bowl to serve.

## Nutrition Amount per serving

Calories  274

Total Fat 20.7g 27% Saturated Fat 14.1g 70%

Cholesterol 51mg  17%

Sodium 266mg 12%

Total Carbohydrate 10.9g 4% Dietary Fiber 3.8g  14%

Total Sugars 2.2g Protein 13.7g

# DESSERTS & DRINKS

## Mix Berry Sorbet

Preparation Time: 10 minutes Cooking Time:

10 minutes

Serve: 1

**Ingredients:**

- ½ cup raspberries, frozen
- ½ cup blackberries, frozen
- 1 tsp liquid stevia
- 6 tbsp water

**Directions:**

1. Add all ingredients into the blender and blend until smooth.
2. Pour blended mixture into the container and place in refrigerator until harden.
3. Serve chilled and enjoy.

**Nutritional Value (Amount per Serving):**

Calories 63

Fat 0.8 g

Carbohydrates 14 g

Sugar 6 g

Protein 1.7 g

Cholesterol 0 mg

# PORK AND BEEF RECIPES

# Mexican Taco

# Casserole

Serves: 3

Prep Time: 35 mins

### Ingredients

- ½ cup cheddar cheese, shredded
- ½ cup low carb salsa
- ½ cup cottage cheese
- 1 pound ground beef
- 1 tablespoon taco seasoning

### Directions

Preheat the oven to 4250F and lightly grease a baking dish.

Mix together the taco seasoning and ground beef in a bowl.

Stir in the cottage cheese, salsa and cheddar cheese.

Transfer the ground beef mixture to the baking dish and top with cheese mixture. Bake for about 25 minutes and remove from the oven to serve warm.

### Nutrition Amount per serving

Calories  432

Total Fat 20.4g 26% Saturated Fat 10g 50% Cholesterol 165mg  55%

Sodium 526mg   23%

Total Carbohydrate 3.2g 1% Dietary Fiber 0g  0%

Total Sugars 1.6g Protein 56.4g

# BREAKFAST RECIPES

## Low Carb Cereal

Serves: 2

Prep Time: 25 mins

### Ingredients

- 2 tablespoons flaxseeds
- ¼ cup almonds, slivered
- 1 tablespoon chia seeds
- 1½ cups almond milk, unsweetened
- 10 grams cocoa nibs

### Directions

1. Mix together flaxseeds, almonds, chia seeds and cocoa nibs in a bowl.
2. Top with the almond milk and serve.

### Nutrition Amount per serving

Calories  244

Total Fat 20.6g 26% Saturated Fat 10.4g 52%

Cholesterol 0mg  0%

Sodium 11mg  0%

Total Carbohydrate 9.8g  4%

Dietary Fiber 6.5g 23% Total Sugars 1.9g Protein 6.5g

# SEAFOOD RECIPES

## Sour Fish with Herbed Butter

Serves: 3

Prep Time: 45 mins

### Ingredients

- 2 tablespoons herbed butter
- 3 cod fillets
- 1 tablespoon vinegar
- Salt and black pepper, to taste
- ½ tablespoon lemon pepper seasoning

### Directions

1. Preheat the oven to 3750F and grease a baking tray.
2. Mix together cod fillets, vinegar, lemon pepper seasoning, salt and black pepper in a bowl.
3. Marinate for about 3 hours and then arrange on the baking tray.
4. Transfer into the oven and bake for about 30 minutes.
5. Remove from the oven and serve with herbed butter.

## Nutrition Amount per serving

Calories  234

Total Fat 11.8g 15% Saturated Fat 2.4g 12%

Cholesterol 77mg  26%

Sodium 119mg   5%

Total Carbohydrate 0.4g 0% Dietary Fiber 0g  0%

Total Sugars 0.1g Protein 31.5g

# Broccoli Gratin

Serves: 4

Prep Time: 35 mins

## Ingredients

- 2 oz. salted butter, for frying

- 5 oz. parmesan cheese, shredded

- 20 oz. broccoli, in florets

- 2 tablespoons Dijon mustard

- ¾ cup crème fraiche

## Directions

➢ Preheat the oven to 4000F and grease a baking dish lightly.

➢ Heat half the butter in a pan on medium low heat and add chopped broccoli.

➢ Sauté for about 5 minutes and transfer to the baking dish.

➢ Mix the rest of the butter with Dijon mustard and crème fraiche.

➢ Pour this mixture in the baking dish and top with parmesan cheese.

➢ Transfer to the oven and bake for about 18 minutes.

➢ Dish out to a bowl and serve hot.

# Nutrition Amount per serving

Calories  338

Total Fat 27.4g 35% Saturated Fat 12.4g 62% Cholesterol 56mg  19%

Sodium 546mg   24%

Total Carbohydrate 11.1g 4% Dietary Fiber 4g  14%

Total Sugars 2.5g Protein 16.2g

# CHICKEN AND POULTRY RECIPES

## Caprese Chicken

Serves: 4

Prep Time: 30 mins

### Ingredients

- 1 pound chicken breasts, boneless and skinless
- ¼ cup balsamic vinegar
- 1 tablespoon extra-virgin olive oil
- Kosher salt and black pepper, to taste
- 4 mozzarella cheese slices

### Directions

1. Season the chicken with salt and black pepper.
2. Heat olive oil in a skillet over medium heat and cook chicken for about 5 minutes on each side.
3. Stir in the balsamic vinegar and cook for about 2 minutes.
4. Add mozzarella cheese slices and cook for about 2 minutes until melted.
5. Dish out in a plate and serve hot.

**Nutrition Amount per serving**

Calories  329

Total Fat 16.9g 22% Saturated Fat 5.8g 29%

Cholesterol 116mg  39%

Sodium 268mg   12%

Total Carbohydrate 1.1g 0% Dietary Fiber 0g  0%

Total Sugars 0.1g Protein 40.8g

# Stuffed Whole Chicken

Serves: 6

Prep Time: 1 hour 15 mins

## Ingredients

- 1 cup mozzarella cheese
- 4 garlic cloves, peeled
- 1 (2 pound) whole chicken, cleaned, pat dried
- Salt and black pepper, to taste
- 2 tablespoons fresh lemon juice

## Directions

1. Preheat the oven to 3600F and grease a baking dish.
2. Season the chicken with salt and black pepper.
3. Stuff the chicken cavity with garlic cloves and mozzarella cheese.
4. Transfer the chicken to oven on the baking dish and drizzle with lemon juice.
5. Bake for about 1 hour and remove from the oven to serve.

## Nutrition Amount per serving

Calories  305

Total Fat 12.1g 15% Saturated Fat 3.6g 18%

Cholesterol 137mg  46%

Sodium 160mg 7%

Total Carbohydrate 1g 0% Dietary Fiber 0.1g 0%

Total Sugars 0.1g

Protein 45.2g

# BREAKFAST RECIPES

# Healthy Breakfast Granola

Total Time: 15 minutes Serves: 5

**Ingredients:**

- 1 cup walnuts, diced
- 1 cup unsweetened coconut flakes
- 1 cup sliced almonds
- 2 tbsp coconut oil, melted
- 4 packets Splenda
- 2 tsp cinnamon

**Directions:**

1. Preheat the oven to 375 F/ 190 C.
2. Spray a baking tray with cooking spray and set aside.
3. Add all ingredients into the medium bowl and toss well.
4. Spread bowl mixture on a prepared baking tray and bake in preheated oven for 10 minutes.
5. Serve and enjoy.

**Nutritional Value (Amount per Serving): Calories 458; Fat 42.5 g; Carbohydrates 37g; Sugar 2.7 g; Protein 11.7 g; Cholesterol 0 mg;**

# Keto Porridge

Total Time: 10 minutes Serves: 1

**Ingredients:**

- ½ tsp vanilla extract
- ¼ tsp granulated stevia
- 1 tbsp chia seeds
- 1 tbsp flaxseed meal
- 2 tbsp unsweetened shredded coconut
- 2 tbsp almond flour
- 2 tbsp hemp hearts
- ½ cup water
- Pinch of salt

**Directions:**

1. Add all ingredients except vanilla extract to a saucepan and heat over low heat until thickened.
2. Stir well and serve warm.

**Nutritional Value (Amount per Serving): Calories 370; Fat 30.2 g; Carbohydrates 12.8 g; Sugar 1.9 g; Protein 13.5 g; Cholesterol 0 mg;**

# LUNCH RECIPES

## Coconut Curry

Total Time: 30 minutes Serves: 4

### Ingredients:

- 1/2 cup coconut cream
- 1/4 medium onion, sliced
- 2 tsp soy sauce
- 1 tsp ginger, minced
- 1 tsp garlic, minced
- 4 tbsp coconut oil
- 2 cups spinach
- 1 cup broccoli florets
- 1 tbsp red curry past

### Directions:

1. Heat coconut oil in a saucepan over medium-high heat.
2. Add onion in a pan and cook until softened. Add garlic sauté for a minute.
3. Turn heat to medium-low and add broccoli and stir well.
4. Once broccoli is cooked then add curry paste and stir for 1 minute.
5. Add spinach over the top of broccoli and cook until

wilted.

6. Add ginger, soy sauce, and coconut cream and stir well. Simmer for 10 minutes.

7. Stir well and serve.

**Nutritional Value (Amount per Serving): Calories 219; Fat 22.1 g; Carbohydrates 5.9 g; Sugar 1.8 g; Protein 2.1 g; Cholesterol 0 mg;**

# Avocado Mint Soup

Total Time: 10 minutes Serves: 2

**Ingredients:**

- 1 medium avocado, peeled, pitted, and cut into pieces
- 1 cup coconut milk
- 2 romaine lettuce leaves
- 20 fresh mint leaves
- 1 tbsp fresh lime juice
- 1/8 tsp salt

**Directions:**

1. Add all ingredients into the blender and blend until smooth. Soup should be thick not as a puree.
2. Pour into the serving bowls and place in the refrigerator for 10 minutes.
3. Stir well and serve chilled.

**Nutritional Value (Amount per Serving): Calories 268; Fat 25.6 g; Carbohydrates 10.2 g; Sugar 0.6 g; Protein 2.7 g; Cholesterol 0 mg;**

# DINNER RECIPES

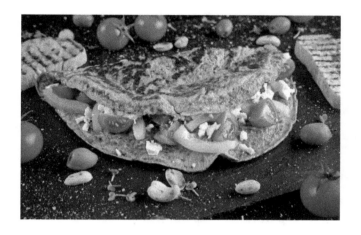

# Spicy Jalapeno

# Brussels sprouts

Total Time: 15 minutes Serves: 4

### Ingredients:

- 1 lb Brussels sprouts
- 1 medium onion, chopped
- 1 tbsp olive oil jalapeno pepper, seeded and chopped
- Pepper
- Salt

### Directions:

- Heat olive oil in a pan over medium heat.
- Add onion and jalapeno in the pan and sauté until softened.
- Add Brussels sprouts and stir until golden brown, about 10 minutes.
- Season with pepper and salt.
- Serve and enjoy.

**Nutritional Value (Amount per Serving): Calories 91; Fat 3.9 g; Carbohydrates 13.1**g; Sugar 3.7 g; Protein 4.2 g; Cholesterol 0 mg;

# Sage Pecan

# Cauliflower

Total Time: 40 minutes Serves: 6

**Ingredients:**

- 1 large cauliflower head, cut into florets
- 1/2 tsp dried thyme
- 1/2 tsp poultry seasoning
- 1/4 cup olive oil
- 2 garlic clove, minced
- 1/4 cup pecans, chopped
- 2 tbsp parsley, chopped
- 1/2 tsp ground sage
- 1/4 cup celery, chopped
- 1 onion, sliced
- 1/4 tsp black pepper
- 1 tsp sea salt

**Directions:**

1. Preheat the oven to 450 F/ 232 C.
2. Spray a baking tray with cooking spray and set aside.
3. In a large bowl, mix together cauliflower, thyme, poultry seasoning, olive oil, garlic, celery, sage, onions, pepper, and salt.
4. Spread mixture on a baking tray and roast in preheated

oven for 15 minutes.

5.  Add pecans and parsley and stir well. Roast for 10-15 minutes more.

6.  Serve and enjoy.

**Nutritional Value (Amount per Serving): Calories 118; Fat 8.6 g; Carbohydrates 9.9** g; Sugar 4.2 g; Protein 3.1 g; Cholesterol 0 mg;

# DESSERT
# RECIPES

## Chocó Chia Pudding

Total Time: 10 minutes Serves: 6

**Ingredients:**

- 2 1/2 cups coconut milk
- 2 scoops stevia extract powder
- 6 tbsp cocoa powder
- 1/2 cup chia seeds
- 1/2 tsp vanilla extract
- 1/8 cup xylitol
- 1/8 tsp salt

**Directions:**

1. Add all ingredients into the blender and blend until smooth.
2. Pour mixture into the glass container and place in refrigerator.
3. Serve chilled and enjoy.

**Nutritional Value (Amount per Serving): Calories 259; Fat 25.4 g; Carbohydrates 10.2 g; Sugar 3.5 g; Protein 3.8 g; Cholesterol 0 mg;**

# Smooth Chocolate Mousse

Total Time: 10 minutes Serves: 2

## Ingredients:

- 1/2 tsp cinnamon
- 3 tbsp unsweetened cocoa powder
- 1 cup creamed coconut milk
- 10 drops liquid stevia

## Directions:

1. Place coconut milk can in the refrigerator for overnight; it should get thick and the solids separate from water.
2. Transfer thick part into the large mixing bowl without water.
3. Add remaining ingredients to the bowl and whip with electric mixer until smooth.
4. Serve and enjoy.

**Nutritional Value (Amount per Serving): Calories 296; Fat 29.7 g; Carbohydrates 11.5 g; Sugar 4.2 g; Protein 4.4 g; Cholesterol 0 mg;**

# BREAKFAST RECIPES

# Blueberry Muffins

Get your antioxidant and energy filled fat boost from these moist and delicious muffins.

Total Prep & Cooking Time: 30 minutes Level: Beginner

Makes: 6 Muffins

Protein: 7 grams Net Carbs: 3 grams Fat:

19 grams

Sugar: 2 grams

Calories: 217

## What you need:

- 1/3 cup blueberries
- 3/4 tsp baking powder, gluten-free
- 1 1/4 cup almond flour, blanched
- 2 1/2 tbs coconut oil, melted
- 1/4 cup Erythritol sweetener, granulated
- 2 1/2 tbs almond milk, unsweetened
- 1/8 tsp salt
- 2 large eggs
- 1/4 tsp vanilla extract, sugar-free

## Steps:

1. Set the stove to heat at 350° Fahrenheit. Use baking or non-stick muffin liners to layer the cupcake cups.

2. In a big dish, blend the Erythritol, baking powder, salt, and almond flour until combined.

3. Whisk in the almond milk, eggs, melted coconut oil, and vanilla extract until a creamy consistency.

4. Carefully stir the blueberries in the batter with a rubber scraper.

5. Evenly empty into the baking cups and heat for 20 minutes.

6. Enjoy immediately.

*Variation Tips:*

1. If you have a nut allergy, substitute the almond flour for sunflower seed meal, just know the muffins may have a slight green tint.

2. You can use either fresh or frozen blueberries. If you opt for the frozen, do not thaw them ahead of time.

# LUNCH RECIPES

# Turkey Burger

# Patties

You do not have to give up having heart healthy burgers while choosing to live a better life.

Total Prep & Cooking Time: 30 minutes Level: Beginner

Makes: 4 Patties

Protein: 11 grams Net Carbs: 1 gram Fat: 8 grams

Sugar: 1 gram

Calories: 117

**What you need:**

- 1/2 tsp oregano seasoning
- 3 tsp olive oil
- 1/2 tsp basil seasoning
- 8 oz. zucchini, grated
- 1/4 tsp salt
- 8 oz. ground turkey, lean
- 1/8 tsp red pepper flakes
- 1 clove garlic, minced
- 1/8 tsp pepper
- 1 tsp parsley seasoning
- 1/4 tsp onion powder

**Steps:**

1. In a large dish, blend the ground turkey, oregano, basil, zucchini, salt, red pepper, garlic, parsley, pepper, and onion powder until completely combined.

2. Divide the meat into 4 sections and create patties by hand.

3. Using a large skillet, heat olive oil. Once the skillet is hot, transfer the patties to the fry for approximately 5 minutes and then flip to the other side.

4. Fry for an additional 5 minutes until

cooked fully.

5. Serve warm and enjoy!

# DINNER RECIPES

# Walnut Chili

You will find that this chili is full of flavor with a couple of secret ingredients that make it stand out from the standard bowl you are used to.

Total Prep & Cooking Time: 45 minutes Level: Beginner

Makes: 4 Helpings

Protein: 10 grams Net Carbs: 5.6 grams Fat:

13 grams

Sugar: 1 gram

Calories: 410

**What you need:**

- 1 tbs extra virgin olive oil
- 2 carrots, diced finely
- 1 tbs ground cinnamon
- 3 stalks celery, diced finely
- 1 tbs ground cumin
- 3 cloves garlic, minced
- 1 1/2 tsp paprika powder
- 2 large chipotle peppers, minced
- 1 1/2 cups walnuts, raw and minced
- 2 bell peppers, diced finely

- 1 1/2 oz. dark chocolate, unsweetened and chopped finely
- 30 oz. tomatoes, diced
- 1/4 tsp salt
- 2 1/2 cups tomato sauce
- 30 oz. black soybeans drained and rinsed
- 1/8 tsp pepper

## Steps:

1. Using a large saucepan, liquefy the olive oil and combine the carrot and

   celery for approximately 4 minutes.
2. Blend the cumin, paprika, garlic, and cinnamon, stirring consistently for about 2 minutes.
3. Finally, combine the bell peppers, chipotle, tomato sauce, soy beans, walnuts, and tomatoes, stirring until fully incorporated.
4. Reduce the temperature to simmer for about 20 minutes or until the vegetables are fully cooked.
5. Melt the chocolate in the chili along with the pepper and salt.
6. Serve while still hot and enjoy!

## Variation Tips:

1. If you prefer spicy chili, add between 1 and 2 teaspoons of cayenne pepper.
2. You can garnish your chili with avocado, cilantro leaves or sliced radishes to mix this recipe up.

# SNACK
# RECIPES

# Chicken Tenders

Move over chicken nuggets! These are a much more improved alternative to your childhood snack.

Total Prep & Cooking Time: 20 minutes Level: Beginner

Makes: 2 Helpings (3 tenders per serving) Protein: 26 grams

Net Carbs: 0.7 grams Fat: 9 grams

Sugar: 0 grams

Calories: 220

**What you need:**

- 1/2 cup coconut oil

- 8 oz. chicken breast tenderloins

- 1 tsp pepper, separated

- 8 oz. almond flour

- 1 tsp salt, separated

- 4 oz. heavy whipping cream

- 1 large egg

**Steps:**

1. In a large dish, blend the egg and heavy whipping cream with the 1/2 teaspoon of pepper and 1/2 teaspoon of salt.

2. Soak the chicken pieces in the blend for

approximately 10 minutes.

3. Using a skillet, melt the coconut oil.

4. Pour the almond flour onto a small bowl and season with the remaining 1/2 teaspoon of pepper and 1/2 teaspoon of salt.

5. Remove the individual pieces of chicken and coat both sides with the almond flour. Set a 13 x 9-inch glass dish to the side.

6. Transfer the chicken to the hot coconut oil and fry for approximately 3 minutes on the side.

7. Serve hot and enjoy!

## Baking Tip:

1. You can also bake these in the oven if you wish. Set the stove to 425° Fahrenheit and prepare a flat sheet with a heavy coating of olive oil. Follow the steps for breading the chicken tenders and place on the prepped sheet. Heat for 10 minutes, flip them and continue to heat for another 10 mins. Note: they will not be as crispy as when they are fried.

# UNUSUAL DELICIOUS MEAL RECIPES

## Shrimp and Grits

This Southern tradition is a staple that can now be enjoyed on the Keto diet with this rendition of cauliflower grits.

Total Prep & Cooking Time: 40 minutes

**Level: Beginner**

Makes: 4 Helpings

Protein: 4 grams

Net Carbs: 5.3 grams Fat: 11 gramsSugar: 1 gram

Calories: 207

**What you need:**

*For the topping:*

- 16 oz. large shrimp, peeled and deveined
- 3 teaspoon butter
- 1/2 tsp thyme seasoning
- 2 cloves garlic, minced
- 1/4 tsp cayenne pepper
- 2 tsp paprika powder
- 1/4 tsp salt

**For the grits:**

**Steps:**

1. Heat the cauliflower in a large pot with the water. Once the water begins to boil, cover with a lid and set a timer for 20 minutes.

2. Check the cauliflower with a fork to ensure it is cooked thoroughly.

3. Drain the water from the pot and transfer the cauliflower to a food blender.

4. Combine the nutritional yeast, salt, butter and almond to the blender and pulse for approximately 2 minutes until the consistency is very smooth.

5. Combine paprika powder, cayenne pepper, garlic and thyme, and in a small dish and whisk to integrate.

6. Combine the mixed spices in a skillet along with the hot coconut oil.

7. Detach the tails and eliminate the moisture from the shrimp by dabbing with a paper towel.

8. Brown the shrimp for approximately 9 minutes while occasionally stirring.

9. Meanwhile, distribute the grits into a serving bowl and once the shrimp are pink, empty the whole contents of the pan on top of the grits.

### Baking Tip:

You may also use frozen shrimp for this recipe. Ensure they have completely thawed ahead of time and decrease the frying time by 3 minutes.

### Variation Tia

- add a garnish of lemon juice, chives or a splash of hot sauce.

- Ghee will work as a substitute for the butter in this meal.

# KETO DESSERTS RECIPES

## Intermediate: Peanut Butter Bars

Serves: 9

Preparation time: 10 minutes Cooking time: 30 minutes

### Ingredients:

- 2 eggs
- 1 tbsp coconut flour
- ¼ cup almond flour
- ½ cup erythritol
- ½ cup butter softened
- ½ cup peanut butter

### Directions:

1. Spray 9*9-inch baking pan with cooking spray and set aside.
2. In a bowl, beat together butter, eggs, and peanut butter until well combined.
3. Add dry ingredients and mix until a smooth batter is formed.
4. Spread batter evenly in prepared baking pan.
5. Bake at 350 F/ 180 C for 30 minutes.

6. Slice and serve.

Per Serving: Net Carbs: 2.8g; Calories: 213; Total Fat: 20.2g; Saturated Fat: 8.6g

Protein: 5.8g; Carbs: 4.5g; Fiber: 1.7g; Sugar: 1.7g; Fat 85% / Protein 10% / Carbs 5%

# Flavorful

# Strawberry Cream

# Pie

Serves: 10

Preparation time: 10 minutes Cooking time: 10 minutes

## Ingredients:

- 1 cup almond flour
- ¼ cup butter, melted
- 8 oz cream cheese, softened
- ½ cup erythritol
- ½ cup fresh strawberries
- ¾ cup heavy whipping cream

## Directions:

1. In a bowl, mix together almond flour and melted butter.
2. Spread almond flour mixture into the pie dish evenly.
3. Add strawberries in a blender and blend until a smooth puree is formed.
4. Add strawberry puree in a large bowl.
5. Add remaining ingredients in a bowl and whisk until thick.
6. Transfer Strawberry cream mixture onto the pie crust and spread evenly.

7. Place in refrigerator for 2 hours.

8. Slice and serve.

Per Serving: Net Carbs: 2.5g; Calories: 217; Total Fat: 21.5g; Saturated Fat: 10.4g Protein: 4.4g; Carbs: 3.8g; Fiber: 1.3g; Sugar: 0.8g; Fat 88% / Protein 8% / Carbs 4%

# CANDY: BEGINNER

# Raspberry Candy

Serves: 12

Preparation time: 5 minutes Cooking time: 5 minutes

## Ingredients:

- 1/2 cup dried raspberries
- 2 oz cacao butter
- 1/4 cup Swerve
- 1/2 cup coconut oil

## Directions:

1. Melt cacao butter and coconut oil in a saucepan over low heat.
2. Remove saucepan pan from heat.
3. Grind the raspberries in a blender.
4. Add swerve and ground raspberries to the saucepan and stir well.
5. Pour mixture into the silicone candy molds and refrigerate until set.
6. Serve and enjoy.

Per Serving: Net Carbs: 0.4g; Calories: 125; Total Fat: 13.8g; Saturated Fat: 11.1g

Protein: 0.1g; Carbs: 0.7g; Fiber: 0.3g; Sugar: 0.2g; Fat 98% / Protein 1% / Carbs 1%

# COOKIES: BEGINNER

# Almond Pumpkin

# Cookies

Serves: 27

Preparation time: 10 minutes Cooking time: 25 minutes

## Ingredients:

- 1 egg
- 1 tsp liquid stevia
- 1/2 tsp pumpkin pie spice
- 1/2 cup pumpkin puree
- 2 cups almond flour
- 1/2 tsp baking powder
- 1 tsp vanilla
- 1/2 cup butter

## Directions:

1. Preheat the oven to 300 F/ 150.
2. Spray a baking tray with cooking spray and set aside.
3. In a large bowl, add all ingredients and mix until well combined.
4. Make cookies from mixture and place onto a prepared

baking tray.

5. Bake for 20-25 minutes.

6. Remove cookies from oven and set aside to cool completely.

7. Serve and enjoy.

Per Serving: Net Carbs: 0.2g; Calories: 82 Total Fat: 7.7g; Saturated Fat: 2.5g

Protein: 2.1g; Carbs: 2.2g; Fiber: 1g; Sugar: 0.5g; Fat 87% / Protein 12% / Carbs 1%

# CAKE

# Coconut Lemon Cookies

Serves: 24

Preparation time: 10 minutes Cooking time: 15 minutes

**Ingredients:**

- 4 eggs
- 3/4 cup Swerve
- 4 oz cream cheese
- 1/2 cup butter
- 1 1/2 tsp baking powder
- 1 tbsp lemon peel, grated
- 1 tbsp heavy whipping cream
- 1 tsp lemon extract
- 3/4 cup coconut flour
- Pinch of salt

**Directions:**

1. Preheat the oven to 350 F/ 180 C.
2. Spray a baking tray with cooking spray and set aside.
3. In a bowl, mix together coconut flour, salt, and baking powder. Set aside.

4. In another bowl, add butter, lemon extract, lemon peel, swerve, and cream cheese and beat until well combined.

5. Add eggs one by one and beat until combined.

6. Add whipping cream and stir well to combine.

7. Add coconut flour mixture to the wet mixture and mix until combined.

8. Transfer prepared mixture into the bowl and cover with parchment paper.

9. Place in the refrigerator for 30 minutes.

10. Remove cookie dough from refrigerator and make cookies and place onto a prepared baking tray.

11. Bake for 15 minutes or until lightly brown.

12. Remove from oven and set aside to cool completely.

13. Serve and enjoy.

Per Serving: Net Carbs: 0.5g; Calories: 66; Total Fat: 6.5g; Saturated Fat: 3.9g

Protein: 1.4g; Carbs: 0.7g; Fiber: 0.2g; Sugar: 0.1g; Fat 89% / Protein 9% / Carbs 3%

# Expert: Lemon Cheesecake

Serves: 8

Preparation time: 10 minutes Cooking time: 55 minutes

**Ingredients:**

- 4 eggs
- 18 oz ricotta cheese
- 1 fresh lemon zest
- 2 tbsp swerve
- 1 fresh lemon juice

**Directions:**

1. Preheat the oven to 350 F/ 180 C.
2. Spray cake pan with cooking spray and set aside.
3. In a large bowl, beat ricotta cheese until smooth.
4. Add egg one by one and whisk well.
5. Add lemon juice, lemon zest, and swerve and mix well.
6. Transfer mixture into the prepared cake pan and bake for 50-55 minutes.
7. Remove cake from oven and set aside to cool completely.
8. Place cake in the fridge for 1-2 hours.
9. Slice and serve.

Per Serving: Net Carbs: 4.6g; Calories: 124; Total Fat: 7.3g; Saturated Fat: 3.9g

Protein: 10.2g; Carbs: 4.8g; Fiber: 0.2g; Sugar: 0.7g; Fat 53% / Protein 33% / Carbs 14%

# FROZEN DESSERT: BEGINNER

## Intermediate: Creamy Raspberry Cheesecake Ice Cream

Serves: 8

Preparation time: 10 minutes Cooking time: 30 minutes

### Ingredients:

- 1 tbsp swerve
- 4 oz raspberries
- 1 tsp vanilla
- ½ cup unsweetened almond milk
- 1 ½ cups heavy cream
- ¾ cup Swerve
- 8 oz cream cheese, softened

## Directions:

1. In a large bowl, beat together cream cheese and swerve until smooth.

2. Add vanilla, almond milk, and heavy cream and mix well.

3. Pour ice cream mixture into the ice cream maker and churn according to machine instructions.

4. In a small bowl, mash raspberries. Add 1 tbsp swerve in mashed raspberries and mix well.

5. Add mash raspberry mixture to the ice cream.

6. Serve and enjoy.

Per Serving: Net Carbs: 2.5g; Calories: 188 Total Fat: 18.5g; Saturated Fat: 11.4g

Protein: 2.8g; Carbs: 3.5g; Fiber: 1g; Sugar: 0.8g; Fat 89% / Protein 6% / Carbs 5%

# Sweet Blackberry

# Ice Cream

Serves: 8

Preparation time: 5 minutes Cooking time: 30 minutes

## Ingredients:

- 1 egg yolks
- 1 cup blackberries
- ½ cup erythritol
- 1 ½ cup heavy whipping cream

## Directions:

1. Add all ingredients to the bowl and blend until well combined.

2. Pour ice cream mixture into the ice cream maker and churn ice cream according to the machine instructions.

3. Serve and enjoy.

   Per Serving: Net Carbs: 1.4g; Calories: 92; Total Fat: 9g; Saturated Fat: 5.4g Protein: 1.1g; Carbs: 2.4g; Fiber: 1g; Sugar: 0.9g; Fat 89% / Protein 5% / Carbs 6%

# BREAKFAST
# RECIPES

# Garlic Bread

All out: 12 min Prep: 12 min

Yield: 4 servings

## Nutritional Values:

Calories: 34, Total Fat: 5.1 g, Saturated Fat:

1.3 g, Carbs: 1.5 g, Sugars: 0.3 g, Protein: 1.3 g

## Ingredients

- 2 cloves garlic
- 1/4 cup olive oil
- 1 portion garlic bread
- 1 teaspoon oregano

## Direction

1. Squirt olive oil into a little skillet. Crush the garlic on a slicing board and add it to the olive oil. Warmth until the garlic tans, the evacuate the garlic and pour the oil over the bread. Sprinkle the bread with dried oregano. Spot garlic bread on flame broil and barbecue until.

# Grilled Vegetable Hero

All out: 25 min Prep: 15 min

Cook: 10 min

Yield: 4 servings

## Ingredients

- 1 half quart cherry tomatoes, divided
- 1 yellow ringer pepper, quartered, seeds and ribs evacuated
- 1 red ringer pepper, quartered, seeds and ribs evacuated
- 1 summer squash, cut on the inclination into 1/2-inch pieces
- 1 zucchini squash, cut on the inclination into 1/2-inch pieces
- 1/4 cup extra-virgin olive oil
- Cut into 1/2-inch rings ,1 medium red onion,
- Legitimate salt and crisply ground dark pepper
- 1 teaspoon red pepper chips, or to taste
- 1 (12-inch long) portion Italian bread with sesame seeds
- Lemon Mayo, formula pursues
- 1 (8-ounce) ball new mozzarella, cut
- 1 pack basil leaves

- Lemon Mayo
- 3/4 cups mayonnaise
- 3 cloves garlic, minced
    - 1/2 lemon, zested
    - 1 teaspoon lemon juice
    - Legitimate salt and newly ground dark pepper

### Direction

1. Preheat the flame broil to medium.
2. In a huge bowl, hurl the vegetables with olive oil and season with salt and pepper, to taste. Orchestrate the vegetables on the flame broil, turning every so often, until scorched and delicate, around 10 minutes. Evacuate to a plate and sprinkle with red pepper pieces.
3. Cut the bread down the middle longwise with a serrated blade. Toast the bread on the flame broil Remove the bread and uniformly spread Lemon Mayo on the two sides. Equitably separate the vegetables on the base parts of the bread. Top with the cut mozzarella and a bunch or so of the basil. Spread with the top portion of the bread and secure with toothpicks. Cut into 4 parts and serve.

# LUNCH RECIPES

# Kale Crackers

Servings:20 Nutritional Values:

Calories: 88, Total Fat: 10.2 g, Saturated Fat:

1.5 g, Carbs: 5.4 g, Sugars: 0.4 g, Protein: 4.6 g

## Ingredients:

- 1 cup Coconut Flour
- Black Pepper, to taste
- 3/4 cup Nutritional Yeast
- 1 tsp Chipotle
- 1 cup Ground Flax Seeds, soaked in 1 cup water
- 1 bunch Kale, chopped
- Himalayan Salt, to taste
- 1 tsp Smoked Paprika
- 2 cup Almonds, soaked overnight, drained and rinsed, finely chopped

## Directions:

1. Set aside after lining the parchment paper with the baking sheet.
2. Combine the almonds, coconut flour, nutritional yeast, chipotle, and paprika. Add the kale and mix well.
3. Pour in the flax and water mixture, season with salt and pepper, and knead the dough.

4. Cover the dough with another sheet and roll out the dough. Cut into crackers, place them on the prepared sheet and dehydrate at 290F / 145C for half an hour. Reduce the heat to 245F / 118C and dehydrate the crackers for about 8 hours, flipping halfway through.

# Frankfurter and-

# Vegetable

## Stew

All out: 46 min Prep: 20 min

Cook: 26 min

Yield: 4 servings

Nutritional Values: Calories: 34, Total Fat: 5.1 g, Saturated Fat: 0.3 g, Carbs: 1.5 g, Sugars: 0.3 g, Protein: 1.3 g

### Ingredients

- 3 tablespoons extra-virgin olive oil

- 1 enormous red onion, diced

- 4 cloves garlic, crushed

- 1 tablespoon paprika, in addition to additional for enhancement

- Fit salt

- 3 tablespoons universally handy flour

- 2 parsnips, stripped and cut into enormous lumps

- 14 ounces little red-cleaned or new potatoes (6 to 8), quartered

- 1 tablespoon juice vinegar

- Naturally ground pepper

- 1/2 cup crisp parsley, generally hacked

- 3/4 cup acrid cream

- 6 ounces kielbasa, cut into little lumps

- Dry bread, for serving

- 3 medium carrots, stripped and cut into enormous lumps

## Direction

2. Warmth the olive oil in a Dutch broiler or substantial pot over medium warmth. Include the onion and garlic; cook, mixing once in a while, until delicate and shimmering, around 6 minutes. Include the paprika and 1 teaspoon salt; cook until the oil turns dark red, around 1 minute.

3. Join about portion of the parsley with the acrid cream in a little bowl and season with salt and pepper. Scoop the stew into dishes; top with the rest of the parsley, a bit of herbed acrid cream and a sprinkle of paprika. Present with bread.

# Keto Hot Dog Buns

Cooking time: 45 min Yield: 10 rolls

**Nutrition facts: 29 calories per roll: Carbs 1.5g, fats 2.1g, and 1.3g proteins.**

**Ingredients:**

- 10 oz almond flour
- 1/3 cup psyllium husk powder
- 2 tsp baking powder
- 1 tsp sea salt
- 2 tsp cider vinegar
- 10 oz boiling water
- 3 egg whites

**Steps:**

1. Heat the oven to 175°C.
2. Mix all dry ingredients: almond flour+ psyllium husk powder+ baking powder+ sea salt.
3. Boil the water.
4. Add to dry ingredients: water+ vinegar+ egg whites and whisk. The dough should be soft.
5. Form 10 hot dog buns.
6. Put them on the baking tray covered with the butter paper.
7. Bake for 45 min.
8. Create the stuffing you like and enjoy.

# SNACKS
# RECIPES

# Hazelnut breadstick
# with seeds

Servings: 10

Cooking time: 40 minutes

**Nutrients per one serving: Calories: 88 | Fats: 14 g | Carbs: 2.1 g | Proteins: 15 g**

**Ingredients:**

- ½ cup hazelnut flour
- ½ cup flax flour
- ½ cup pumpkin seeds
- ½ cup sunflower seeds
- 2 eggs

**Cooking process:**

1. You can prepare the dough in the same way as described in the previous recipe.
2. Preheat the oven to 220°C (425°F).
3. In a bowl, beat the eggs by a mixer until dense mass, and add flour and seeds. Mix it all again.
4. Cover the baking sheet with parchment. Lay out the dough.
5. Bake in the oven for 10 minutes. Cut into the desired number of sticks and put on the switched-off oven for 20 minutes.

# Preparation Time: 5 minutes

Cooking Time: 25 min Servings:6

## Nutritional Values:

Fat: 18 g.

Protein: 8 g.

Carbs: 2 g.

## Ingredients:

- 4 Whole Eggs
- ¼ cup Melted Butter
- ½ tsp Salt
- ½ cup Almond Flour
- 1 tsp Italian Spice Mix

## Directions:

1. Preheat oven to 425F.
2. Pulse all ingredients in a blender.
3. Divide batter into a 6-hole muffin tin.
4. Bake for 25 minutes.

# DINNER

# Wednesday:

# Breakfast: Simple

# Egg Salad

Egg butter is a savory, flavorful way to start your day.

**Variation tip: mix in a little fresh dill or chives.**

Prep Time: 5 minutes Cook Time: 10 minutes

Serves 2

**What's in it**

- Eggs (4 qty)
- Butter (5 ounces)
- Kosher salt (.5 tsp.)
- Fresh ground pepper (.25 t)

**How it's made**

1. Place eggs in a large pot and fill to cover with cold, filtered water.
2. Bring to a rolling boil and let cook for 8-minutes.
3. Carefully drain eggs and plunge into a bowl of ice water to stop the eggs from overcooking.
4. After the eggs have cooled, peel and chop.
5. Combine with butter, kosher salt and fresh ground pepper

6. Goes great with lettuce leaves. Also try with avocado slices, smoked salmon, turkey, or ham.


**Net carbs: 1 gram**

Fat: 69 grams

Protein: 12 grams Sugars: None

# Intermediate:

# Almond & Flax

# Crackers

Servings:20-24 crackers

Nutritional Values: Calories: 47.7, Total Fat: 5.2 g, Saturated Fat: 1 g, Carbs: 1.2 g, Sugars: 0.1 g, Protein: 1.9 g

## Ingredients:

- ½ cup Ground Flax Seeds
- ½ cup Almond Flour
- 1 Tbsp Coconut Flour
- 2 Tbsp Shelled Hemp Seeds
- ¼ tsp Fine Sea Salt
- 1 Egg White
- 2 Tbsp Unsalted Butter, melted

## Directions:

1. Preheat your oven to 300F / 150C.
2. Combine the flax, almond, and coconut flour, hemp

seed, and salt. Add the egg and melted butter and mix until well combined.

3. Transfer the dough onto a sheet of parchment paper, cover with another sheet of paper and roll out the dough. Cut into crackers and arrange them on the prepared baking sheet.

4. Bake for half an hour, allow to cool and serve.

# THE KETO LUNCH

# Sunday: Lunch:

# Cheese and

# turkey rollups

**What's in it:**

- 3 slices of turkey lunchmeat
- 3 slices of cheese (your choice)
- ½ avocado
- 3 slices of cucumber
- a quarter cup of blueberries
- handful of almonds

**How it's made:**

1. Using your cheese as bread, make "turkey rolls" by rolling up the turkey meat, a few slices of avocado, and the cucumber slices.
2. Enjoy, and snack on the blueberries and almonds.
3. Contains 13 net carbs.

# KETO AT DINNER

## Sunday: Dinner:

## Lamb Chops

Celebrate Saturday night with juicy lamb chops served with herbal butter. Perfection.

*Variation tip:* serve with a simple green salad or other vegetable. Can also substitute pork chops.

Prep Time: 15 minutes Cook Time: 10 minutes Serves 4

### What's in it

- Lamb chops (8 qty)
- Butter (1 T)
- Extra virgin olive oil (1 T)
- Kosher salt (to taste)
- Fresh ground pepper (to taste)
- Lemon, cut into wedges (1 qty)
- Set chops out to bring to room temperature.
- Sprinkle with kosher salt and fresh ground pepper.
- Heat butter and oil in skillet. Add chops and brown on both sides, 3 to 4 minutes each side.

- Serve with lemon wedges and butter.

**Net carbs: 1 gram**

Fat: 90 grams

Protein: 44 grams

Sugars: 0 gram

CPSIA information can be obtained
at www.ICGtesting.com
Printed in the USA
LVHW011020220221
679517LV00019B/1037